Tales *from the* Tail End

My Cancer Diary

ANANYA MUKHERJEE

Illustrations by Peeyush Sekhsaria

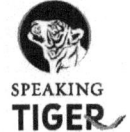

SPEAKING TIGER PUBLISHING PVT. LTD
4381/4, Ansari Road, Daryaganj
New Delhi 110002

First published in Hardback by Speaking Tiger 2019

Copyright © Shantanu Bhasin 2019
Illustrations copyright © Peeyush Sekhsaria 2019

ISBN: 978-93-89231-13-7
eISBN: 978-93-89231-12-0

10 9 8 7 6 5 4 3 2 1

All rights reserved.
No part of this publication may be reproduced, transmitted,
or stored in a retrieval system, in any form or by any means,
electronic, mechanical, photocopying, recording or otherwise,
without the prior permission of the publisher.

This book is sold subject to the condition that it shall not, by
way of trade or otherwise, be lent, resold, hired out, or otherwise
circulated, without the publisher's prior consent, in any form of
binding or cover other than that in which it is published.

Contents

Prologue	7
1. Ki and Ka	13
2. Dukh, Dard and a Season of Hope	15
3. The Breast Has Become Kali	19
4. Women and Scans	21
5. Khuddar and Deewar	23
6. Pyar Kar Le	27
7. It's Time for Self-praise	29
8. Why Women Make Better Leaders	30
9. My Veins Are Like Seasons	34
10. Charitraheen	37
11. What Does a Cancer Patient Dream Of?	40
12. It's Time to Love	43
13. What Should My Well-wishers Bring Me?	46

14. Love: 0, Friendship: 1 — 50
15. Vultures Everywhere — 53
16. Wanted! A Shot in the Arm for the Survivors' Club — 56
17. Tonight I Want to Tell the Best Friend — 59
18. Husband and Conversations — 62
19. Tell Me a Ghost Story — 66
20. Mothers with Malice — 73
21. The Tall Women — 76
22. Like a Banyan Tree — 79
23. Beauty and the Beast — 80
24. Yolo — 85
25. Hope As a Strategy — 88
26. Fear Is Just a Four-letter Word — 91
27. These Legs — 97

Afterthoughts — 99

Prologue

As Ananya wrote these 'tales from the tail end', she cocked a snook at life, its temporality, and the slippery, overestimated virtues that we attribute to people and social norms. She chose to focus on the joie de vivre of life. A lifetime can be lived in a moment, she seems to be saying, and it can be lived utterly wasted even in a whole span. She lived it fully; she laughed at it, challenged it and even in the throes of pain, winked at its ironies. Was she celebrating it or was she mourning it? As she writes her observations on day-to-day things, isn't she saying, 'I am living the moment as the shastras say—dropping many social and moral compunctions attached to it by social pundits.' No long-term plan but the immediate moment, the here and the now was her reality. This is the sad but ultimate truth she dwells on in her writing.

It is difficult to have the right perspective if the object of focus is close to one's heart and the loss of it too recent. The so-called 'object' in this case is Ananya, a persona with multi-hued facets besides the obvious and the outer personal ones. She was a professional par excellence, a wife, daughter, daughter-in-law and a friend and beyond all these interpersonal relationships, she was an individual in her own right, and a strong one.

In a style that is as inimitable as she was, like the tragic hero of a Shakespearean drama, she remains indomitable, tragic but heroic in her writing as she was in life. If life challenged her with cancer she gave it a brave and befitting fight—'Ya, ya, I know death and all'—she seems to be saying. As I read the pages she wrote, I am struck by the fact that she is, she was and she remains irrepressible, not to be subdued and always her own self. The very first song in the book, '*pyar kar le*', sets the tone. It is a promise to meet the ultimate lover at every turn of life, in all the lifetimes to come. She is not worried about the overrated 'life and death' question for it is the moment of love, this very moment that is to be lived. She is living the dream of love, leaving behind the uncertainties of a love life. Every piece is a new version of this song. Go for the essence of the song, she seems to be coaxing the reader—'*pyar kar le ghadi do ghadi*' for you never know when life will betray you. Live the moment!

As she chooses her topics, one notices all of them are the moments as she lives them, the here and the now. There is no past, no future there. She is almost Buddhist in living the moment with its full depth, collateral ironies and laughs on the side at oneself and the world. That brings me to think that intellectually she is capable of grasping the essence of Buddha's teachings, but the kind of immediacy she has in her writings, seems to imply precision and focus in her topics as well as the narrative. She could never stand fools and when life decides to fool her she has an irreverent, happy, tongue-in-cheek response at hand for it. Happiness in her writing implies that which is not happy. That remains the subtext. She does touch on Pablo Neruda in one of her pages that has an undercurrent of sadness. I don't know, but I have a feeling that she must have read these lines where Neruda says,

> *Tonight I can write the saddest lines.*
> *I no longer love her, that's certain, but maybe I love her.*
> *Love is so short, forgetting is so long.*
> *Because through nights like this one I held her in my arms*
> *my soul is not satisfied that it has lost her.*
> *Though this be the last pain that she makes me suffer*
> *and these the last verses that I write for her.*

Living life, living cancer, she is the same girl who would reiterate with Neruda, '*You can cut all the flowers but you cannot keep spring from coming.*' She would mourn the loss of love but celebrate its tenderness in the same breath saying,

> *You and I, Love, together we ratify the silence,*
> *while the sea destroys its perpetual statues,*
> *collapses its towers of wild speed and whiteness:*
> *because in the weavings of those invisible fabrics,*
> *galloping water, incessant sand,*
> *we make the only permanent tenderness.*

So much for the content. Coming to her style, the critic in me finds it well-synchronized with her attitude and to use a rundown expression, 'in sync with her philosophy of life'. She would have surely replaced the expression for she hated clichéd words, expressions, thoughts and way of life *et al*. Sure, the undercurrent of pain, wasted limbs and death are there, but they have been unequivocally denied their claim to a rightful place in the saga of cancer in her life. She adopts a style that is ironic, funny and tragi-comic in tone. Reading the pages, one reads what is unwritten. It's the style that introduces the writer. In her writing, life walks with its chin held high. If death is the adversary, she considers it below her dignity to even engage with it, what to say of conceding defeat. She would rather give life its due by smiling wryly at it.

How does she do it? She juxtaposes megalomaniac life against the threat of a disappearing hairline and the ominous disease cells throbbing in her veins. She chooses the technicolour dreams that come under the effect of morphine drugs rather than the wasted dreams…She devotes a happy chapter to the 'Ka' and the 'Ki' on her windowsill. Striking a dialogue with them, she forgets pain and soars high and light like the pink paper in one of her pieces. The eye shadows take prime space on those rainy days of Mumbai that precede a chemo. These shadows are bright and light and they make one beautiful and ready to be admired. She is in love with people, with friends and with the loved one in her life.

As a missive of hope she had ordered a new table, a lovely sofa, and a couple of sarees and designer blouses she was going to use when the chapter of cancer would finish. Finish it did, leaving behind *Tales from the Tail End*. Life, like love, is short but takes long to forget.

Dr Mridul Bhasin
Jaipur, June 2019

1
Ki and Ka

There are several crows where I am living now temporarily in Mumbai. I spend many a sleepless night looking at the night lights, and fall asleep to the sound of the morning azaan. Just as I am comatose in the early hours of the morning, one particular crow starts cawing insistently at the window. It's not the English-type 'caw', this one's a desi. He goes ka, ka, ka…plaintively, nonstop, loudly.

In my chemo-laden head, I hurl the choicest of abuses at it. Sometimes, I hurl a pillow at the window along with the expletives. *Haramzada*, refuses to budge. Then I think it must be an old ancestor come to pay me a visit. I take a good look at Ka. He has dishevelled hair and knowing black eyes. Convinced he looks familiar, I give him some bread soaked in milk. Ka rolls his beady eyes at me, skirts the bread and steps aside (later, a flock of pigeons feast on it, shit heartily on the windowsill and lay some eggs—they're more likely my ancestors).

Meanwhile, Ka keeps up with his 8 a.m. harassment. Then I realize how similar we are, and begin to soften. In my tattered T-shirt and Bermuda shorts, with hair not knowing whether to start growing or prepare to fall, I'm feeling more Ka these days.

On mornings like today, Ka and I stand at the window, both looking disdainfully at the universe, both waiting to get our Ki back.

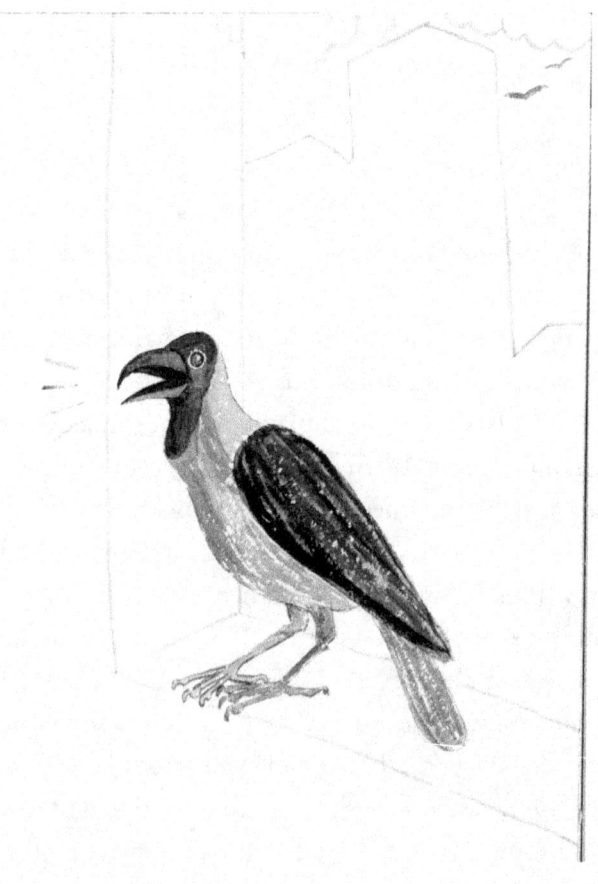

2
Dukh, Dard and a Season of Hope

A few well-meaning folk who visit me hold my hand, weep some, and say they're sorry for me. I don't know what to do, so I pat them gently on the thigh (ladies only) and say, 'Don't worry, it'll all be okay.' They look at me strangely and mumble that I'm strong.

I've always been strong-hearted and proud of it. So am I not sad? When I was first diagnosed with Stage One of an aggressive type of breast cancer, I was stunned and disappointed in myself but quickly found my resolve. I chose to fight cheerfully, selecting the best doctors, eating healthy, praying hard, sending out affirmations to the universe, with a deep belief and faith that I'd be okay.

Then I learnt hope was a bad thing.

A year later, I was told my breast cancer had grown back and metastasised (metastasis is when your cancer has spread from its primary site to the rest of your body; it is also called advanced cancer, and the jury is out on its cure.) I googled it on my phone and to be doubly sure, on my laptop. It said the same thing. Now I became unimaginably sad. But I bit my lip and kept my chin up in front of the traitors (doctors) and the caretakers (family). Like every bad Bollywood film ever, I gulped and told the husband that something had gone into my eye. And then came the waterworks. I cried into the pillow, at the mirror, into the curtain, in the shower and to a few friends who caught me offguard. The rest I avoided. As much as it's important to cry your share, I also believe there's a time to grieve and a time to snap back. Self-pity is a bottomless pit. So now I've crawled

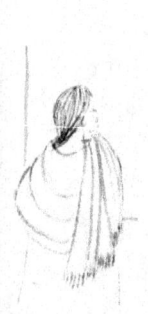
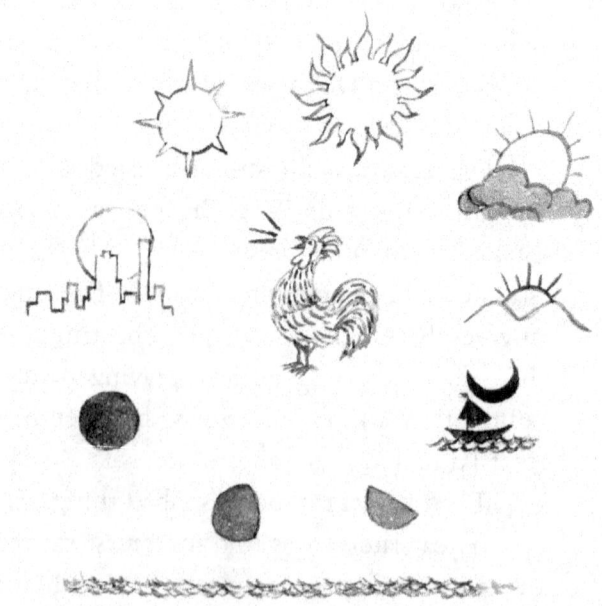

out, and walk noisily around the house with a shawl draped around my shoulders like Rajesh Khanna in *Anand*, scolding the husband and teaching him for the two-hundredth time how to fold a towel correctly, with the right side up. I'm past my Dukh.

Do I have Dard?

Oh yes, of all kinds that come with an illness like this one. But heartbreak and bikini wax still top my list in the 'most painful' charts.

Do I have Hope?

Difficult to say. It's a long answer. The husband says, 'Try starting from the conclusion.' I pretend I haven't heard.

I stay on the nineteenth floor of an apartment in Thane now and though Ka the crow doesn't visit here (quite a long flight from Bandra, with all the planes coming in the way), there's a Crazy Cock down in the slum nearby that crows shrilly all day. For decency's sake, let's call it the Crazy Rooster. I hear his vociferous crowing first at the crack of dawn, then he calls boisterously to the neighbourhood at 10.39 a.m., next I record his loudspeaker-like pitch at 1.21 p.m., then he yells his lungs out at 3 p.m. and so on, all bloody day. Clearly his body clock is screwed. Then I suddenly remember it's spring, my favourite season, a season for craziness and hope. My *sukh-dukh ki saathin*, Neha Khullar, is visiting me. We stand at my bedroom window and look out at the dull blue water of the Thane creek. I tell her that its stillness unnerves me. She listens carefully, then cracks a joke like friends do to distract; I throw my head back and laugh. The sun sets between the brown-green hills and a silver moon rises above the water, just like a watercolour in motion. We stuff our faces with food, giggle into the night and look at the highway traffic till 2 a.m., till Crazy Rooster goes off again.

To be able to breathe, walk noisily, listen to a rooster crowing, scold a husband, laugh with a friend and look at something so beautiful, is in itself a miracle. This time I'm not banking on the hope of a better tomorrow. I'm just glad to have had a beautiful spring day. A day of life is still life!

3
The Breast Has Become Kali

Those who know me well, know that under a superficial veneer of dignity, I've always been flippant and borderline vulgar ('downright cheap' the husband corrects). Well, what to do, this is who I am.

In my head, I've always referred to breasts as 'boobs', a part of the anatomy that was created for physical attraction, for pleasure and joy (I'm the woman equivalent of 'oh boy...cleavage!' and you'll always find me giggling at rack jokes). For me, breasts have never held any more importance than that. When some of my friends became mums and their babies started photobombing them by grabbing their breasts just as the camera clicked, I relegated the breast to a role of motherly comfort; benign and nurturing.

Now I think of the breast as Goddess Kali. And mine gone rogue. Malignant and ravaging through my body in a terrible red rage. Trying to take my life.

Unstoppable by any force. Maybe our aeons-old attitude of patronising the breast, ridiculing it and treating it like an object for pleasure or necessity has finally turned her into an angry marauder.

The breast as Kali demands her rightful respect and dignity. Who knows, only then she might stop her rampage.

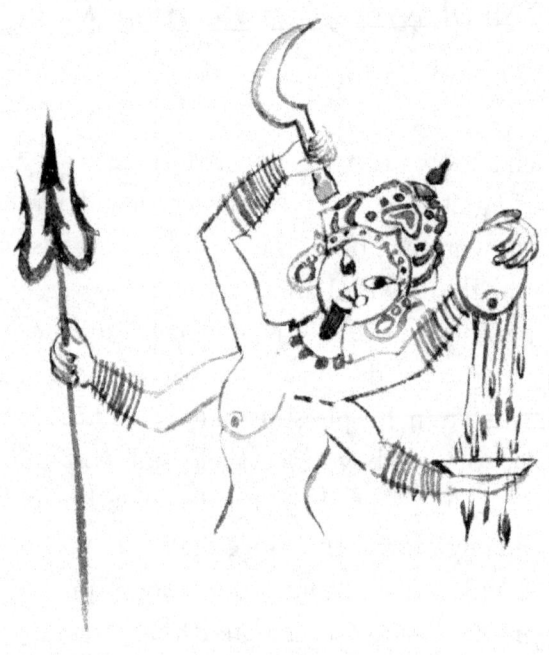

4

Women and Scans

When I queued up for a PET CT scan a few days back, I was pleasantly surprised to find four other women in line. The attendant stuck some needles into us and packed us off to a cold room with strict instructions to keep quiet.

But when Allahabad, Gwalior, Pune, Hyderabad and Kolkata gang up, no amount of shooshing by the attendant could work. Those of us who'd gone into the giant machine's belly before, reassured the first-timers. The conversation then shifted from tumours to hair growth strategies, veered towards healthy recipes and finally settled on an all-time favourite amongst women—saris! (Sabyasachi will feel vindicated finally.) Ombré chiffons, printed georgettes, crisp cottons and soft silks were discussed threadbare in that morning hour.

Finally, when the time came for the giant to swallow

us up one by one and spew us out along with our morbid futures, we went in with a glint in our eyes. I for one thought of the deep magenta Jamdani my mother has recently bought for me for the 2018 pujas. *Inshallah!*

5
Khuddar and Deewar
(not starring Amitabh Bachhan)

In the hospital, I make many acquaintances. We spend several hours chatting about this and that, while getting chemoed, waiting for check-ups, queuing for tests etcetera.

In these exchanges, many a time, my cancer comrades thrust their phones at my face. First, I think they are showing me their shiny new Xiaomi phones. I sing praises wholeheartedly. They give me disappointed looks. So I add an encouraging comment or two about Chinese manufacturing. Then I realise they are trying to show me something else. They are showing me their pre-cancer photos and videos. When they had long hair, or just hair in the case of men. When they wore lipstick or had smart moustaches (some women had them too). Photos of how well, healthy and active they looked. I wonder why they show me their photos when

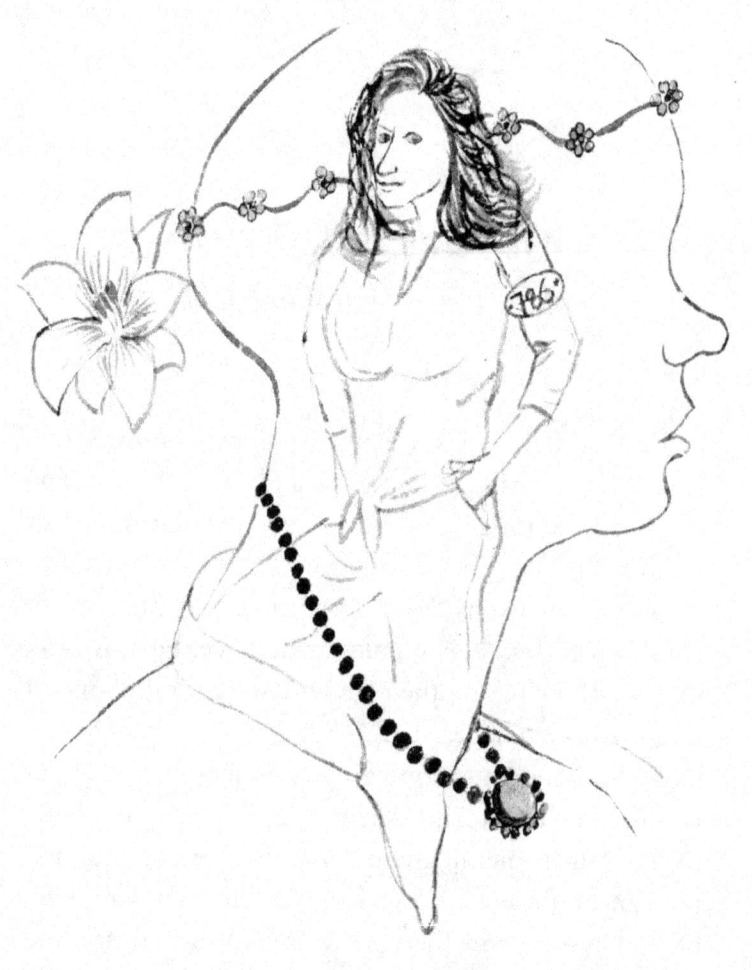

it obviously makes them a shade despondent. Then it strikes me. They are trying to show their past avatars as functional members of society. With hair, eyebrows, jobs, egos and physical strength.

Over time as our physical strength wanes, we become unable to fend for ourselves. Soon, the world starts looking at us as infirm and dependent on doles—physical, emotional and financial. Some think of us secretly as invalids. Some not so secretly. It makes us reconcile to the reality that we need help. It strips us of our egos.

Hence, my comrades carry their photos around. Photos from another lifetime. A family jauntily going off somewhere in a pack. A man laughing heartily, baring his fangs, who now has pipes sticking out of his mouth. A woman beaming confidently at a child's birthday party, complete with messy streamers and a crooked homemade cake, now dependent for basic things like cooking food and taking a bath. A man standing on a hillock in a striped sweater, holding his wife's hand, hands that wheel him around now.

To bridge this dashing past and despondent present, I come up with an idea. The hospital should pin identity cards on us not with photos of us as we are now, but from our past, when we were active and functional. It will help us feel better and improve other people's judgment of us.

Like everyone else, I take time to accept this reality of my various inabilities. I try to run errands, pay bills, file insurance claims, work some and throw some old-time attitude around. When my strength fails, caregivers try to tell me I shouldn't push myself (the husband adds that a toothless person shouldn't think of eating steak). I do a bit of yelling, asking everyone to back off with their alms, and see how well I handle everything. Turns out I am a cat's whiskers no more. I am just airy, penniless, proud and now incapable of managing on my own.

In the end, I buckle down and variously eat crow, humble pie etcetra. But not before rolling my eyes and saying—*'Main aaj bhi pheke hue paise nahi uthata.'*

6
Pyar Kar Le

The eighteenth chemo courses through my veins but my mind is on other important things today. Like Valentine's Day. I remember the flutter of excitement I used to feel in my teens and twenties, and the cynicism of the later years. But today my heart is humming loudly…lines from an old Hindi number (tried to sing too but the day-care nurse glared at me). To my loved ones!

Aaj se apna vaada raha
Hum milenge har ek modh par
Dil ki duniya basaayenge hum
Ghum ki duniya ka darr chhod kar
Jeene marne ki kisko padi?
Pyaar kar le ghadi do ghadi…

From today there is a promise made
We will meet at every turn
We will settle in a world of the heart

Leaving behind the fear of a world of sorrow
Who cares about living or dying?
Love, for a moment or two...

(Listen to it if you haven't, but strict advisory against the video!)

7
It's Time for Self-praise

Once upon a time, a lover had told me, 'Before you, I've never met anyone with real pink lips.' I had immediately gloated, and thought vaingloriously of my peaches and cream complexion for a long time after. Now the mirror looks back at me with ashen lips, sallow complexion and sunken eyes.

'What do I have, then?' I ask.

'A sick person's pallor,' the husband says helpfully. I give my trademark cold stare and he goes back to his mobile game. Suddenly I think of my smile, and smile. It can still light up a room. Not like chandeliers anymore, no, and not a large room by any means, but in the company of that smile you won't be groping in the dark for sure.

8
Why Women Make Better Leaders

It's 8th March, I tell the husband, and try to strike up a conversation on why women make better leaders. I haven't even reached mid-sentence when he tells me that the doctor says I will get well sooner if I spoke less. Dejected, I turn the monologue inward. The problem with having a conversation with your rich inner self is you can never stay on track, you jump from one thing to another and before you know it, you are astray. Like I am.

I am already thinking of how little girls grow up. I start thinking of two of my friends who I've seen over a decade grow into successful, confident, talented and secure women. My mind is filled with images of the rag-tag, gentle and eager-to-please Garima Wahal from college with whom I would sing love songs on drunken nights and who would always hold my hand tightly while crossing the road. She's now a very talented, super-confident and much sought-after Bollywood professional. Now my mind jumps to an address in South Delhi that can instill fear in the bravest of the brave—'Masjid Maut' (may have been Masjid Moth). There lived bravely the first five-digit earner I knew, Deepakshi Jha, who was super smart, super fun, super resourceful and always fed random hungry friends of friends. She continues to be all these, while juggling a high-profile career now. I write about them because over the course of my illness, I've spent considerable time parked at their homes while they've gone about their business. And I'm always impressed by how perfectly their homes run on auto-pilot. They manage pressing careers, (pressing) in-laws, homes and babies, and I don't mean effortlessly like superwomen. They invest themselves fully in their home and work relationships, deal with bumps and disappointments with courage and handle their duties with elan. They are sharp as tacks, highly focused, work hard as hell and yet keep an eye out for a friend in distress, hear out a colleague going through heartbreak and offer practical assistance to the needy. It's unfortunate that our social construct demands men to be unidimensional and single-minded whereas women juggle multiple roles. However, it is this challenge that a lot of women are able to turn into an opportunity for their own growth and those around. But I'm digressing again.

Back to the homes of these two, where I while away productive days having engaging discussions with myself. I find their housekeepers, drivers, staff, and if I run into them, their work colleagues, a content and happy lot. One of their *andawalas* told me how ma'am loaned him money in a crisis, in lieu of eggs (creative!) and now doesn't even remember to take free eggs (to preserve his ego and earnings, presumably). Another's housekeeper let out gently that didi not only gave her money to put a roof over her head in distress but also gave her *bartans* so she could start cooking right away (sound practical help!). They are just a couple of examples I've witnessed firsthand. Countless women

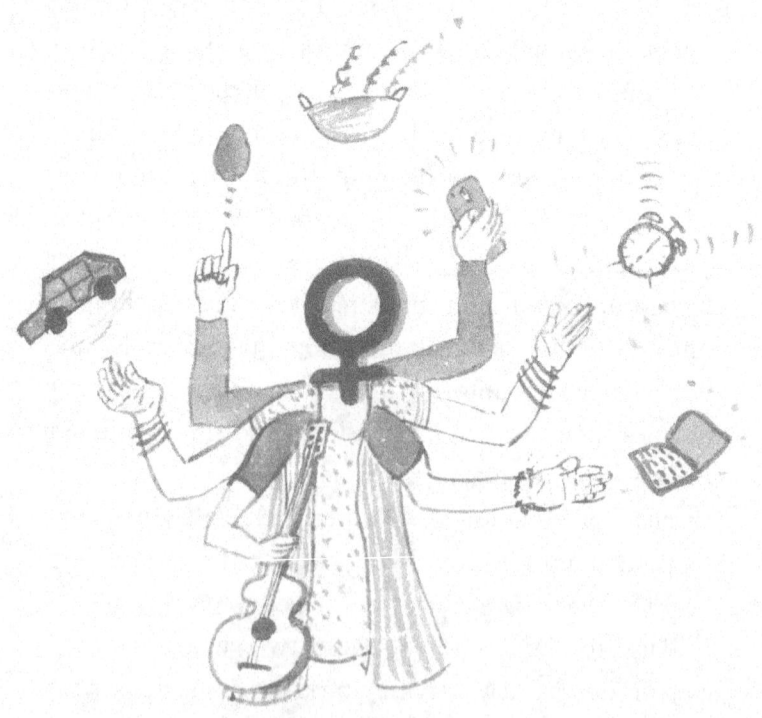

are acing this role of keeping their kitchen fires burning while extending themselves to touch the lives of those around them.

And that's when I get my answer. Women make more well-rounded leaders and managers because the one ingredient that completes skill, determination, creativity, intellect and hard work is Compassion. An invisible golden thread that holds it all together, richly, beautifully.

Happy Women's Day.

9

My Veins Are Like Seasons

After my lymph node surgery last year, my left hand had been declared out of bounds for any further pricks and cuts. While in the hospital, they always tie a red plastic band around it that says 'No procedure'. While this pleases the left hand quite, the right one sulks as this means it has to bear the brunt of all kinds of pricks (like literally ☺).

The poor right has to deal with weekly blood tests, regular injections and six-hour-long chemo sessions, fearing which the veins decide to hide each time before a session begins. Not to be outdone, two solid nurses work up a war strategy to draw out the veins. One belts the arm up tightly with a tourniquet, the other one grabs the wrist, and together they start slapping all over like perverts, trying to arouse the veins. The veins know better, they slide further under the skin. A battle of wills ensues between the two parties, and at the end, an expert third nurse joins in. This one has seen enough in life to know that grabbing and slapping don't always work, nor does love. She takes a deep breath, opens her Third Eye, invokes her animal spirit and jabs the needle somewhere. With full confidence. It miraculously hits the target, some blood squirts back into the syringe. This sight pleases the three witches. They smile at each other in satisfaction and give a mental high five. All this while I calmly study the ceiling, looking for dust in the air conditioner vents.

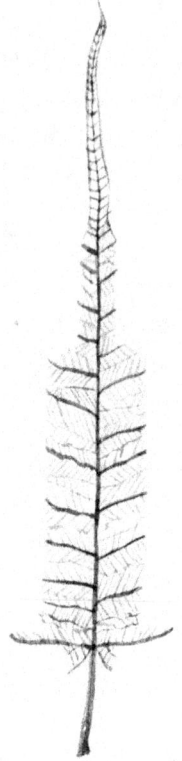

For my staring at the ceiling and not kicking the nurses, the veins decide to show me their colours later. The first few days after the offensive, they turn red and angry like summer, scorching my arm day and night, breathing fire should anything touch them. A few days later, they turn sad, swollen and green like the monsoon, ready to burst out at the slightest. More days pass; the green veins turn into a beautiful autumnal yellow, with tinges of pale orange on the inside of the arm. Thereafter, like in a hard winter, they shrivel up and throb, demanding ice packs and cold gels. The painful winter lasts a while but before I know, them damn veins are feeling better again. They are not raging with summer's fury, weeping with monsoon's misery or turning an autumn gold anymore. Like spring they've plumped up, ready for a fresh onslaught.

10

Charitraheen

As I start losing hair the first time round, I try to be cool and sport a bald pate. I forget I am no Lisa Ray, I can't pull it off. I look like a boiled white egg. Neighbourhood aunties look at me pitifully. Passersby stop in their tracks. Children stare at me like they've seen a ghost. And men, who would earlier stare at the breasts while talking, now stare at the breast and the scalp while talking. I get distracted. Then I buy a wig—a human hair one that costs five digits. I remember to reduce one while telling the husband its price. He is happy. His world is an old, familiar and cheap place. Like his night pajamas, frayed at the edges, permanently yellowed and a hundred years old.

Since she is a human hair wig, she has a mind of her own. She covers me well on most days, sitting snug, as if she were my very own hair. Then she turns moody and hangs limp over my ears, as evident as a plastic wig.

In summer, as I pretend to be cool, she makes me hot under the collar. When it's humid, she puffs up and rises like a freshly baked cake.

When my chips are down, I hang her up on a hook by the window. There she stays, pretending to be mellow, pretending to be sad for me, gently swaying in the breeze, all the while looking longingly at the world outside. Aching to adorn someone else's egghead, I presume. Someone more exciting. Maybe a film star gone bald or someone in that category.

Soon, I get well and toupee her up again for my appearance into the world. She's unreliable as ever. Turns slippery when it rains. Becomes dodgy when I tilt my head back to admire the clouds. I am mortified she'll expose me in public like in a bad dream. She doesn't. Just when I start trusting her, she refuses to settle down on important hair days. As much as I pat her down, she resists being docile. Eventually, I make peace with her unpredictability.

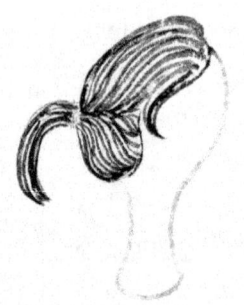 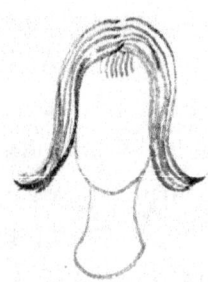 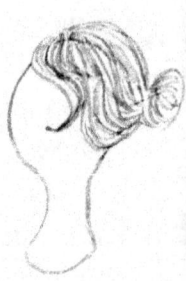

Her character continues to be indiscernible. Sometimes she is ramrod straight, at times curled up, mostly she swings in between.

My wig. You are like me. Headstrong, fancy-free, unreliable and charitraheen.

11

What Does a Cancer Patient Dream Of?

I could say I dream of zombies of other cancer comrades I meet along the way, but I would be just dramatising for effect.

I have always been a vivid dreamer and for years I had a recurrent dream of missing vehicles—trains, buses and planes. The story lines were always messy, I was making a scramble for a train but there was no coach with the number printed on my ticket or my train was slowly chugging out of the station while I was running on the platform drenched in sweat (I was neither Kareena Kapoor, nor did any Shahrukh Khan-type hand emerge out of the train lovingly even in my dreams—such has been my confidence level). Other times, I dreamt anxiously of planes I was about to miss while my suitcase just wouldn't close or my partner went for a dump at the airport with my boarding card and never showed up (now I think the only explanation could be he was embarrassed after using up my card as toilet paper).

No such thing ever happened in real life. In my waking hours, I continued to be one of those hyper annoying Bengali travellers who reach the station or airport at high noon for a night journey, doublecheck tickets always, hang clothes and lock bags a night before, keep boarding passes clutched close to the chest like family jewels (and also wear a monkey cap anywhere under twenty-five degrees, the husband adds uninvited).

Well, moving on, a year into my cancer treatment, I again started dreaming of journeys. But this time I had to mostly cross dark waters, navigate unknown spaces or walk across badly dug up roads with mud, silt and dust flying all around and the destination was almost always unknown. I have never woken up distressed from these dreams, I have always been intrigued. Besides some of these dreams had my loved ones in them, so no worries there (at least for me).

Then the doctors put me on morphine tablets for pain relief and though there's no documented evidence, narcotic drugs are often known to cause strange or hallucinatory dreams. My own became larger than life. Bigger canvasses, bizarre settings, technicolour effects and heightened drama. I dreamt of crossing several feet high, deep green, silky waves against iridescent skies; gliding down a thirty-feet escalator in the dark but with a familiar hand holding mine securely; cycling in a yellow meadow as huge as the universe, with someone yelling behind me in a happy booming voice, 'Hey! can you hear the sonic?'; hanging on the sides of a rickety bus like a bat in the night, amidst random people, travelling on an unknown route, the driver dropping us somewhere midway and the voices of some passengers echoing, 'If you just cross these green waters you'll reach Pakistan' (I'm sure going to hell). Crazy like that!

But not all dreams are dark, crazed or in unfamiliar territory. Why, the other night I dreamt of the boss giving me feedback that both the quality and speed of my work was poor and in need of urgent improvement. I woke up feeling normal. In other good dream nights, I enjoy lovely parties with warm, glamorous people, sipping on some fine whiskies or guzzling beer on a moonlit beach with friends and singing Rabindra Sangeet; gently flowing words, dresses and hair (in my dreams I still have it).

Last night I dreamt of my very good, very beautiful (and very rich) friend, Nitika. Whenever she'd visit Jaipur from Delhi, she'd buy half of Amrapali's jewels. I saw us shopping together and for every piece she was buying, I was getting two of them! The only mistake I made was in telling the husband about my dream the morning after. He said he preferred the ones where I was crossing over dark green waters to Pakistan. And wished Nitika would continue her Jaipur visits for better pursuits than Amrapali.

12

It's Time to Love

While picking eye shadows at Sephora today, a line plays in my head: 'We are most alive when we are in love.' Someone great, whose name eludes me now, has said this. With one foot firmly planted on a banana peel and the other one headed God-knows-where, I wonder if this is the opportune time for self-love? Or any kind of love? Or to dream in colour? Or to even feel good?

Last evening: Standing in the balcony at dusk, I look at the sky turn a sorbet yellow, bringing with it a cooling thunderstorm. The wind lifts up a bright pink paper bag that floats, turning round and round in circles, nineteen floors up, towards me. Birds overhead fly thick and fast homewards. Within minutes, the sky comes down in a grey-black dome and it starts pouring. Children in the slum nearby start dancing. The rain and its antics cool my soul. And up my heartbeat with desire. I check myself out. With never-ending chemotherapy and a general breakdown in all things beautiful or desirable, I should have more gravitas, more depth. Instead, I feel lightheaded like the pink paper bag. I feel alive. And in love.

This morning: I wake up with the faint smell of rain and snatches of a beautiful dream that I don't remember fully. I arrange my sparse hair carefully over my shiny scalp and take a taxi to meet friends at a mall. The rain-drenched streets are full of good-looking strangers and lovers walking hand-in-hand. On cue from the universe, a song from the film *Life in a Metro* plays—

> *Berang si hai badi zindagi, kuch rang toh bharo*
> *Main apni tanhaayi ke vaastay ab kuch toh karoon*
> *Jab miley thodi fursat, khud se kar le mohabbat*
> *In dinon, dil mera, mujh se hai keh raha,*
> *Tu khwaab saja, tu jee le zara*
> *Hai tujhe bhi ijaazat, kar le tu bhi mohabbat…*

This life is so colourless; fill some colour in it
I must do something now for my loneliness
When there is time to spare, fall in love with yourself
These days, my heart, it keeps saying to me:
You create dreams, you live a little
You too have permission; you too can love…

Broken or maimed by life; with a future or hair or without either; it's always a good time to love.

To dream in colour. To feel alive. Bring on the eye shadows!

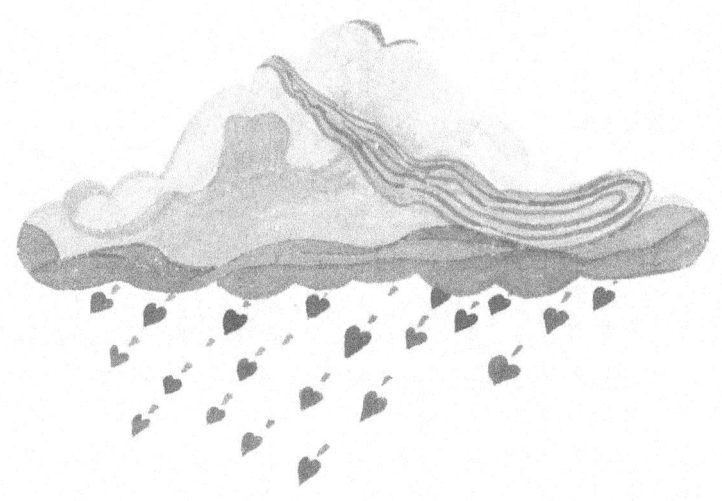

13
What Should My Well-wishers Bring Me?

I'm forever grateful to my well-wishers and friends who send or bring me wonderful things. Yellow lilies brighten up my room, a bag of fruit brightens up my mother's mood, there's a silk stole that I drape around my arms now and then (even in this heat), just to feel beautiful, and a Dove gift hamper which when opened, filled the room magically with the sweet smell of *ek chauthayi* milk, and ever since I told another pal that I've stopped reading serious books, he thoughtfully gets me a stack of *Cosmopolitan* and *Filmfare* magazines, which I read cover to cover, to stay on top of the latest bedroom moves and Taimur Ali Khan's airport looks. In this indulgent phase, I wonder what else I should ask my well-wishers to send me?

1. A fuzzy little feeling: Prolonged illness can make your soul dull. The weekly needles, the drab hospital colours, the bitterness in the mouth, the blank eyes of fellow cancer comrades…everything adds up to the growing dullness in the heart. As a counter, I have suddenly started enjoying everything that makes me feel warm and fuzzy. My friends' babies gurgling, throwing spit balls in the air, trying to eat their own hands and legs and opening their toothless mouths to show off their brand new pink tongues, warm the cockles of my heart. As much as sloppy dogs, smiling with all forty-two teeth, goofing around, making a fool of themselves, makes me happy on many a prickly day.

2. Your children's art: While my interest in horizontal, helpless babies is fairly recent, I have always been fond of the vertical ones. Ones who can run, tell you their names when they are lost in a mall, ask for food when they are hungry and can point where it hurts. These little ones are usually a delight, more so when you don't have to take them home with you. And I've always swelled with the pride of an aunt and the delight of a teacher when my friend's or relative's children make art. I've pored thoughtfully over li'l Ishaan's crayon drawing for me, wondering if the sun is squinting because it's hot and if our heart really is a balloon; while little Kian's spirited narration of an enoooormous monsterrrr had me engrossed. Keep them coming!

3. Sell me some dreams: I've never been sold on dreams and have always patted myself for being hardcore practical. But now when I can't walk for fifteen minutes without getting tired, I want someone to tell me that

I can make that road trip to Jaisalmer, through bumpy, dusty roads where a wrong turn can lead to nowhere. When my lonely heart aches, I need to believe I'll be able to do that gondola ride in Venice under a bright blue sky, floating over water that's like green silk, an occasional window flashing a bunch of red roses while a thousand blossoms bloom in my heart. When I call a colleague and hear they're out for lunch, I dream of rushing out with my work mates to the nearest biryani joint, laughing at some inside joke, flinging my bag hurriedly over my shoulder, heels clicking. More than anytime ever, I need makebelieve now.

4. *Tell me a good story*: I'm a sucker for stories. When not looking out the window and sighing, my mother reads me some contemporary Bangla short stories from a big fat library book. These are stories of unrequited love, family dramas with a twist, crimes of passion and tales of the unexplained. I carefully follow her mouth, spilling out the words, lest I miss something. Before I know, I take centrestage in these dramas, fighting for the underdogs, siding with the protagonists, crying for the fallen and sighing with my mother, when the stories end abruptly. So if you have a story to tell, I'm all ears!

5. *Macherjhol*: At my core is a *hangla bheto bangali* (greedy, rice-eating Bong) always aching for a good fish curry. After my surgery last year, a close friend from Pune, went straight to the market, bought fish, cooked it and drove a hundred and fifty kilometres, bringing with him a piping hot *pabdajhol* and some fried *rui*. Not

a drop spilled on the way and every drop nourished my soul. The memory of that afternoon still lingers—drowsy and sated with fish and rice, the indignities of surgery forgotten, we had looked at the monsoon clouds gathering in the distance and chattered away all afternoon.

As my list comes to a close, the husband quips, 'You have forgotten the most important thing.' To my wide-eyed stare he says, 'Money. Ask everyone to bring you some money, along with fish curry or dreams or whatever else they're getting.'

Point noted, sir.

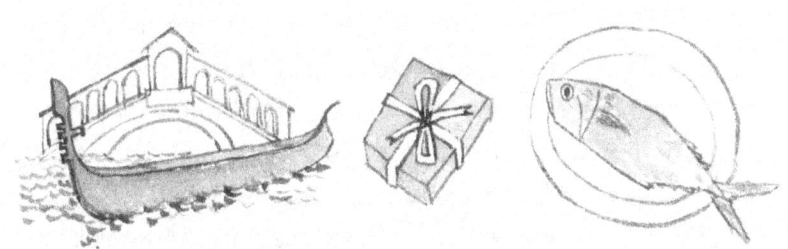

14
Love: 0, Friendship: 1

My Kishore Kumar playlist springs to life with the melodious and heady *rimjhim gire sawan* and even though the bright blue sky blazes outside, I think dreamily of heavy rains beating against a distant window, a head on a shoulder, a heart brimming with love and eyes brimming with the knowledge that this is what it will always be. Some window, some song, always a reverse countdown of the hours and forever unrequited.

People spend an entire life looking for that one perfect love, always unattainable, and hot in its pursuit, climbing its highs and falling into its lows, turn blind to the soothing, balm-like love of friends. For its histrionics, its theatrical value, the way it messes with our brain and hormones, and the constant fear of it running out, love is seen as a higher emotion, while friendship quietly pulls along in its slipstream.

Love: 0, Frienship: 1

In the last couple of weeks, in between bouts of fever, pain and bedridden days, my most favourite friends decided to drop in. They brought with them food for the stomach and hyacinths for the soul. First the girls descended in a burst of energy, shaking me out of my gloom, feeding me, dressing me up in bright lipstick and whisking me off to a pub on a Saturday night, reminding me of what used to be my watering hole all these years. Instead of feeling out of place, I sat delighted, sipping on a hot chocolate, listening to old rock, watching beautiful people drink, dance and make merry! And when my back started hurting sitting on those fancy backless benches, one of the girls offered her back as a back rest and the other one gave me a heavenly massage back home.

Next, my boys visited, calling me dudette like old times, looking at me rather sensitively behind their charming jokes and uproarious laughter. They took me for a quiet drive to the nearby creek, where we spent several *'zindagi na milegi dobara'* moments, looking back at life, our long pauses broken by the gurgling water and the gushing wind. I regret that I broke the spell by pointing to a naked fisherman nearby, with six-pack abs, soaping himself vigorously and the boys that they are, they got easily distracted.

After they returned me home, I wiped off the lipstick, kept the sunglasses back in the box, put away the good clothes, climbed into my sick bed and turned straight to page No. 63 of Ruskin Bond's *Book of Simple*

Living. It says, 'Nothing really ends happily ever after, but if you come to terms with your own isolation, then paradoxically, it becomes immediately possible to find a friend. And friendship is also love.'

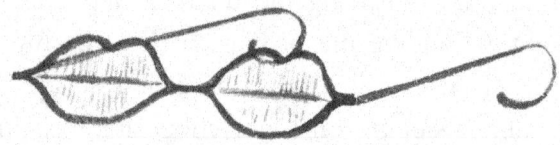

Experiments with Simple living & High Thinking

15
Vultures Everywhere

Trapped at home while it pours outside, I learn about the survey findings of Thomson Reuters that ranks India as the world's most dangerous country for women, ahead of Afghanistan, Syria and Saudi Arabia. It has stirred a hornet's nest, with anyone who's anyone rejecting the report, calling the findings alarmist and sensationalist. The rejecters are crying hoarse that we cannot top the charts over countries where women are not even allowed to speak, drive, participate in public life etcetera.

What they effectively mean is India has come a long way. As Indian women, our danger rating should be downgraded from endangered (earlier) to vulnerable (now). Vulnerable to gruesome rapes, mild molestations, frequent trafficking, sundry beatings, revenge stripping, punishment burnings, lighter gropings, ambiguous sexual harassments and such. So how can we be no country for women?

Involuntarily, I am taken back to one of my earlier biopsies done at a hospital, which is not my regular one. After completing the biopsy and sweet-talking through it, the middle-aged male doctor traced his fingers on my forehead, nose and cheeks, and said, 'You are a beautiful girl. You should WhatsApp me. I will help you through this phase.'

Lying down face up, my first thought was to spit in his eye or elbow him with my one good hand. My second thought was to stay quiet and let it pass. Usual choices. A vague incident, difficult to constitute as harassment, the learned would say. Definitely not enough to make us a land dangerous for women.

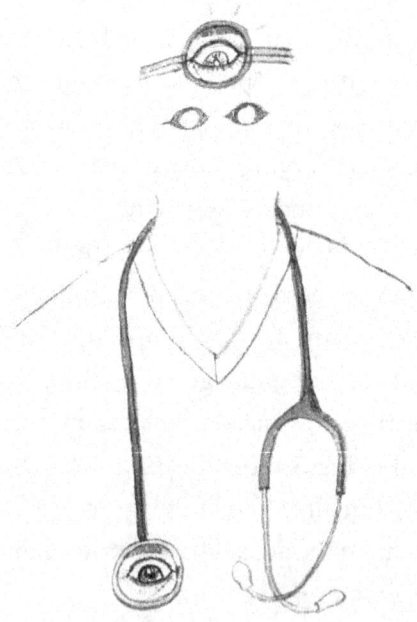

Vultures Everywhere

At other times, I have caught ward boys, attendants, random men probably related to patients, peep through an accidental gap in the curtains or a sudden opening of the door while I was being examined. I often wondered who these men were, who would get excited by cancerous breasts.

Now I look at the rain falling over a wasteland and think of vultures, with their exceptionally sharp sense of smell. A sense that helps them spot the sick, the wounded and the dead. Smells that turn them on. Smells of easy targets.

It is understandable that being judged as a country most dangerous for women is an affront to our national pride and the collective conscience of our civilized, empowered society. Next time, the researchers should call out the perpetrators instead. Such as—'Research finds Indian men are the most dangerous in the world'.

16
Wanted! A Shot in the Arm for the Survivors' Club

Someone recently complained in a cancer-related blog about the term 'survivor' used for patients who didn't kick the bucket (or haven't just yet). Why not a cardiac survivor or a diabetes survivor, the gentleman hotly protested. I think probably survivors are those that manage to live through a catastrophe. Like rape, acid attack, cancer or a violent storm. Despite being life-threatening, a heart attack or diabetes doesn't have the associated drama to be classified catastrophic.

In any case, even I grudge the term 'survivor'. It has a hollow ring to it. Like someone has cleaned out your insides but has left you with just enough to limp through life. I wonder who is worst hit by a storm? One who gets blown away, heroic in suffering, witnessed by all, glorified in being the sure-shot victim, the grateful dead? Or the almost-victims, ones who didn't make the cut? Who weathered the storm and lived to tell the tale of shards from that fateful time?

And what do you get after you survive a storm? Admission to the Survivors' Club? Where you have to dole out sugar-coated bitterness to prove a lame point? That you fought hard because you had no choice? Heaven won't have you and hell here won't let you go.

What do you get by putting your survivorship on display, peddling it daily, keeping it relevant? TED talks? Giving goosebumps to your audience as they listen to you in awe, and maybe wipe an occasional tear and then go back to their normal lives, admiring you highly, but secretly relieved that they are neither a victim nor a survivor; while you, already a discard now, go back to your silent suffering night, trying to make peace with your missing life and limbs? So much for the benefits of being a member of the said club!

Maybe survivors' clubs were popular in an earlier time that belonged to moral science books. Applauding bravery in distress, setting examples for others and issuing war cries in capital letters like 'DON'T LET WHAT YOU CAN'T DO, STOP YOU FROM WHAT YOU CAN DO!'

But I tell you this sentiment won't last much longer. We demand better incentivisation. More compensation from life. We need to reinvent the survivors' club and make it less depressing. No more becoming a living version of inspirational talks. Throw in some goodies—

money, free sex, an enjoyable vice, something outrageous, spectacular and exclusive. Think survivor million-dollar lotteries. Sponsored round-the-world-trip (with free medical support). Decadent parties. Survivor Tinder. Special invitation to the mile-high club. The works.

Let us brim over, for once.

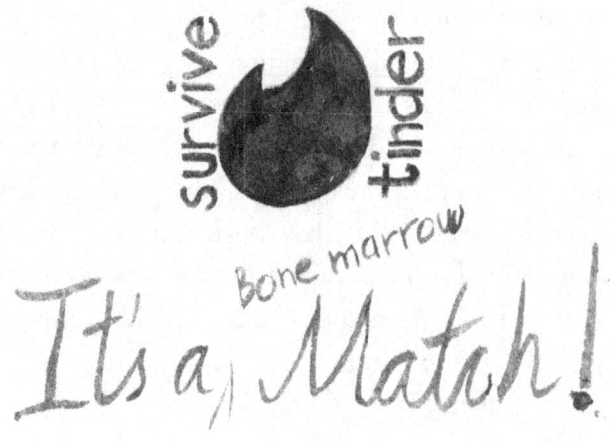

17
Tonight I Want to Tell the Best Friend

First they take me out to fancy dinners and dances. Then they make long conversations into starry nights. Afterwards, I am indulged with elaborate and utterly unviable life plans.

Even after cancer strikes, some romance continues to dribble. Enthusiastic after-getting-well dreams are laid down and talked up. Some compassion tugs at their hearts or loins (whichever is deprived at the time), and I continue to be at the receiving end of affection.

Then in the aftermath of prolonged illness, I am dropped. Aftermath—after the mathematics has been done. I am slipped out from the mainstream. Made irrelevant for my non-participation in everyday life. In its rigours, joys, sorrows, sexiness and dailiness. I am incapable of being fancied any more. Or made long-range plans with.

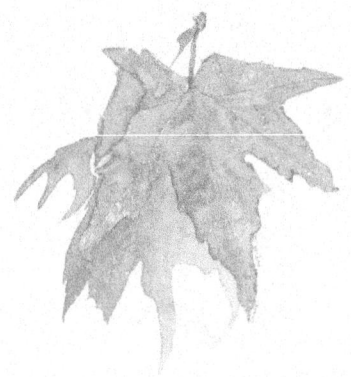

I am dropped but not discarded completely. (They are god-fearing people with an irrational fear of karma or what they think it is. Memories and affections are different things altogether. They are clever, they know for these there is no higher appellate.) So now they engage me in cursory health discussions. Encourage me to take up duties more in sync with my affliction. 'Keep company with other ailing or retired people'. 'Join support groups'. 'Crusade for a cause'. 'Meditate'. (Or paint on glass to remain calm.) The message is—stay coiled and sedated.

But how do I douse the fire that rages on in my heart?

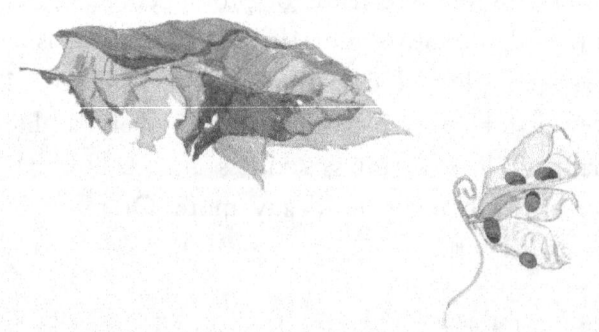

Tonight I Want to Tell the Best Friend 61

I remember an ongoing conversation with the best friend for many years now. Love is the world's oldest and most well-orchestrated con job, I always told her. She told me I had hardened up. I didn't mope on being turned down. I didn't yearn in spring. I didn't sigh at poetry. I didn't hang on to lovers' coat-tails. I could just sit with my hands folded on my lap and bide my time for people to return or go to hell.

'You have turned into an Old Goddess,' she had gently accused. 'Clever and demanding blood; unruffled and detached.'

Tonight, I want to tell the best friend that I'm no Old Goddess.

Tonight, my heart is broken by the world that has moved on.

Tonight, I lick my wounds in solitude.

Tonight, I think of Neruda and his saddest lines.

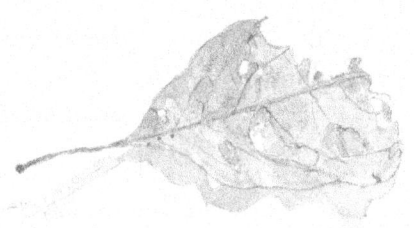

18
Husband and Conversations

Though I would have liked the subject to be Husbands and Conversations, yet it has to be singular for the time being.

With my treatment on in Mumbai and the incumbent's hometown being in Jaipur, we spend long periods of separation leading to a highly happy relationship. We also spend an inordinate amount of time talking on the phone, on subjects other than—can you press my shirt, find my wallet, give me food, fetch me water, get my phone, switch on the light, switch off the AC, switch on the AC, switch off the light….

Away from the tedium of domesticity, we indulge in refreshed conversations where he drops many pearls of wisdom, while I manage to gather some.

About God: I share how I am inundated with suggestions on rituals to cure me. They range from getting *mahamrityun jai jaap* done, feeding black dogs on Thursdays, cows (on all days), to not feeding myself on special days reserved for gods. All this ostensibly to appease the Almighty and instill fear in the power of His wrath. The husband says that if He is the creator of the Universe and the Supreme Almighty, He better not look for petty appeasements and indulge in random anger when bhakts end up eating eggs on Tuesday. If God exists, he must be bigger than that. Food for thought.

About Death: In our long-distance relationship, we often touch unappetizing subjects like death. I tell him I am not sure if I am scared of dying, though I don't like the idea of it very much. We talk of funny movies like *Hangover 2* and *3 Idiots*, where a person's ashes in a jar is a matter of much jesting. The husband says probably that is the best way to look at it. Everyone who lands here, however fancy or plain, stinking rich or generally stinking, with an abundance of close human relations or only cats for occasional company, will end up in a lidded jar only to be immersed or spread somewhere. No exceptions there.

About Love: 'Everyone loves differently. Just because your vision of love doesn't match with mine, doesn't mean I love you any less,' he says. I nod in comprehension and add thoughtfully, 'It's like—one man's love is another man's porn.' From the sound of it, it seems like the husband has slapped his forehead dramatically. Then he hangs up. I wonder why?

Love Again: We are all diehard romantics at heart. Thus, most of the love (or lack thereof) that we give or receive is nothing more than an expression of romanticism. Real love goes deeper than that. It is far more enduring. It is less pleasing and comforting, but harder and real. It is a lot like being grounded, while romance is about flying high. 'Hmm,' I say gravely. 'True love is like a hard mattress. Tough in the short run, good for the back in the long run.' He speaks in a wonder-filled voice, 'You may not be the brightest bulb in the chandelier, but you do light up sometimes.' I am not sure if it's a compliment or an insult. It must be the hard mattress stuff.

Finding Happiness: is an unrealistic goal. Happiness is not a mountain you manage to climb one fine day and plant a flag on. You can't grasp happiness. Or store it in a jar to whiff morning, noon and night. It is short-lived, occasional, transient. And heartbreaking when you lose it. Peace and contentment are more attainable goals. Once you achieve them, they stay with you. They even sound good to the ears.

Apart from these valuable learnings, I also glean some essential life hacks from the husband:

1. The power of telepathy: can close cupboards, make wet towels lift themselves up from the bed and stretch themselves on the clothesline to dry. It can also command water bottles to arrive promptly by the bedside.

2. Gifting made easier: Birthdays, anniversaries and special occasions deserve warm handshakes, best wishes and sometimes a light hug. All other gifts are meaningless.

Husband and Conversations

3. Mastering multi-tasking: Listening to your spouse talk endlessly while playing a challenging game on the mobile can be mastered with ease. You just need to pay attention to the last part of any sentence, as you may be asked to repeat.

4. Sleeping is an evolved art: It takes years of practice to be able to sleep anywhere, anytime and growing a crocodile's skin to ignore the verbal jibes and poking in the ribs by the wife. Once you have mastered it, you will be rewarded with dreams of daisies when you sleep productively day after day while the grass grows tall under your feet.

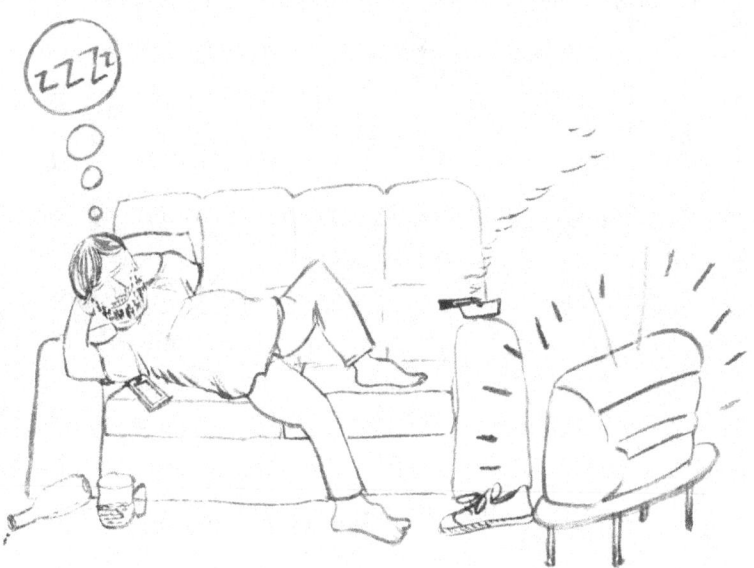

19
Tell Me a Ghost Story

In the month of July it rains non-stop in Mumbai. In tandem, in the month of July, the family complains non-stop about the rains in Mumbai. For a change of scene, I drag them to Igatpuri near Nashik to a monsoon resort. The husband leaves for his hometown, Jaipur, but not before calling me chemo-brained. 'Who in their right mind goes to a monsoon destination to escape the monsoon?'

Turns out, this is the first time he is right in all our married years. In Igatpuri, the rain is intense, cold and tiresome. We spend the days cooped up in the hotel room, watching the rain fall copiously. The family complains variously—about the dampness, the grey skies, the knee aches, the food, no streaming of Bangla channels (a Maharashtrian conspiracy, they say), the dim lights in the room and the overall gloom.

The only thing that pleases everyone is the view.

The suite has French windows that open out into a balcony with breathtaking views of the verdant Western Ghats. The hills are dotted with trees, each a different shade of green. Through the centre of the mountains, a stream of water comes gushing down. On the left, another small stream meanders zig-zag before trickling down and getting lost in the greens. Cutting through the range goes the central line of Indian Railways. Rain-drenched trains snake through the day, whistling melodiously at the ghats and sometimes disappear into the smoke of the waterfalls.

On this day after breakfast, my grandmother and I have parked ourselves on the easy chairs in the balcony to escape the whining parents. My father is complaining that there is never enough light in these fancy hotels and it hinders his Sudoku-solving. My mother is watching the day's breaking news about an air-hostess' apparent suicide. The channel is dramatizing it with a deathly background score and lurid graphics.

'The voyeurism of our times,' I tell my grandmother and she sighs.

My grandmother looks exactly like how she has looked, ever since I was born. Thin, yellowish fair and tall, in an off-white sari draped in the fashion Bengali women did a century back. Her sari is always messy and unkempt. She constantly chews paan or betel nuts, her hands are rough and scaly but she has always had an abundance of affection, especially for me. When I was small, I used to find great comfort in the soft folds of

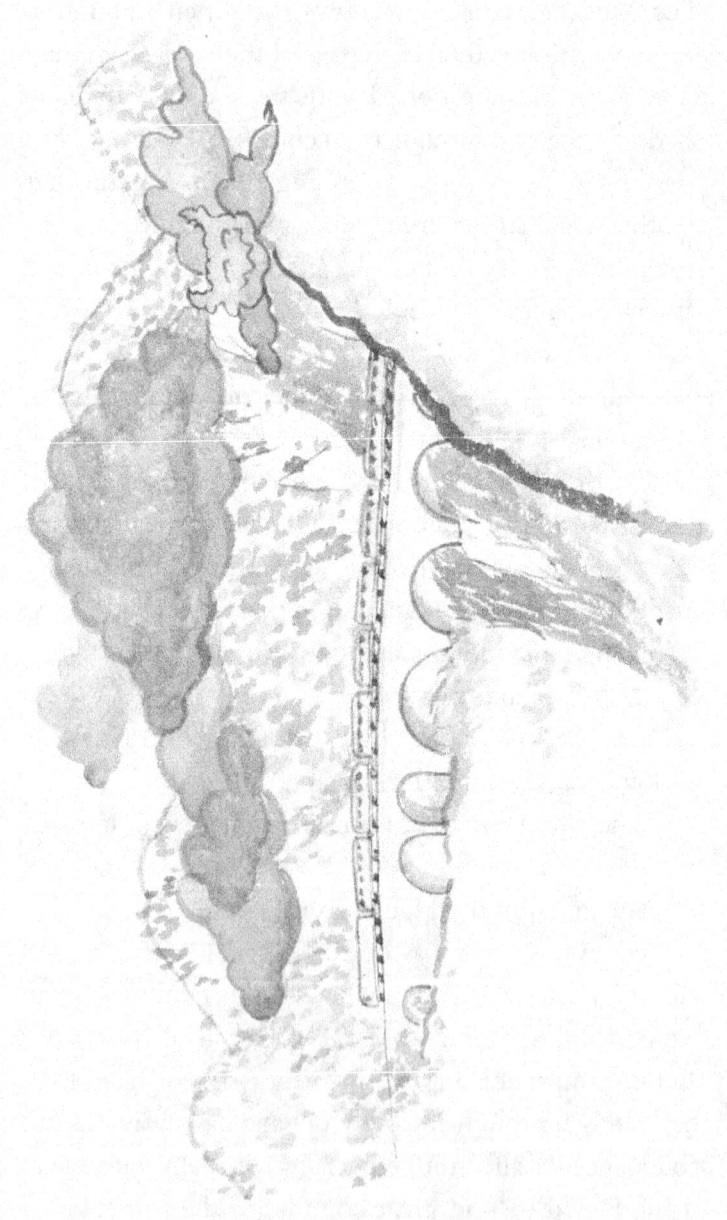

her soiled sari, smelling paan, picking crumbs of nuts and nestling against the warmth of her yellowish skin. (As I grew older, I started frowning upon the same unkemptness).

Presently, she opens her quaint silver paan box, takes out her nut-cutter and deftly starts slicing betel nuts without even looking.

'I want you to leave me your paan box, after you… you know,' I say.

She gives me a wan smile that seems to say, who knows who's going first. Her sarcasm doesn't please me much and grandmother-granddaughter continue to watch the hills in silence.

Soon a thick layer of mist glides over the hills and momentarily we can see nothing except the swarm of clouds.

'Papa…ghost, Papa…ghost,' a small child in the adjoining balcony yells pointing at the clouds. Papa looks at us and drags the child back into their room. A long mournful cry of an Alco engine cuts through the mist and slowly the clouds scatter away. A wispy ball of cotton, shaped like a question mark remains. It has escaped the thick cloud and now hangs solitarily in front of the mountain.

'Tell me a ghost story,' I say to my grandmother. She stuffs a paan in her cheek and starts promptly.

'This one time your grandfather was very sick after a bout of pneumonia and the doctors had almost given up on him. I was quite young and your mother must have been in school. We lived in our old ancestral, joint-family home with its four-poster bed by the window. The window had thick black grills, wooden shutters and a wide parapet, on which one could sit comfortably. Since it was a large family, I had a lot of household work. Someone or the other would be by your grandfather's side all day, tending to him, while I did my share of chores. Late at night, I would return to our room exhausted, ask your grandfather if he needed anything, and then after pulling up his covers, making him warm and comfortable, I used to take out the rolled-up mattress from under the bed and go to sleep. I presumably did this because I wanted your grandfather to be comfortable on the bed.

'Now you must remember that your grandfather was orphaned at a young age and I had never met his parents. But on this night, I had a lucid dream. I saw a stout woman with a thick nose a lot like your grandfather's, sitting at the window, holding the window grill with one hand and looking at me with angry eyes. I got scared and asked her who she was and what she wanted. The apparition said in a hoarse voice, "Your mother didn't groom you well, so I had to come to teach you a few things. Listen, when someone close to you is very sick, you should stay by their side and sleep with them. You should touch them gently with your hands often, soothe them, pat them and channel your positive energies into them. A loved one's touch has healing energies that can cure." Saying this, the spectre stretched her legs on the parapet, asked me to make her a paan, chewed it at leisure and only then disappeared through the grills.

'The next morning, I rushed to tell the elderly women of the house about my dream, and they readily confirmed that indeed the description of my aggressive nightly visitor fitted my mother-in-law. From that day on, I took my position again on the four-poster bed, pressing your grandfather's feet, rubbing his back, keeping my hand lightly on his arm as he slept. With time, he healed. I don't know if it worked but these days they call it Reiki or energy healing or something like that.'

'It is a good story,' I acknowledge.

My grandmother smiled, held out her rough scaly hand with yellowed nails and patted my arm gently. She kept rubbing her coarse palm on my arm for quite a while. It felt like I was back in the folds of her sari, with its sharp, fresh smell of paan, while she kept patting me gently, absentmindedly.

I woke up sometime later to the shrill, complaining whistle of a train. I watched it roll by the mountain. Then I turned my head and looked inside through the glass. My father was sitting under the lone light bulb and going at his Sudoku with a pleasant frown. My mother was sitting on the edge of the bed, intently following the suicide story, which had progressed fast and was now being touted as a murder.

If my grandmother was alive today she would have been over ninety-five.

With insomnia and restlessness characterizing my nights ever since I have taken ill, I am condemned to sleeping alone on most days. Now I think I have company. Of the vivid memory of that rough hand gently patting my arm. I don't know if it will heal me. It certainly soothes me.

20

Mothers with Malice

One of the perks of my illness, I had hoped, would be sweet, gentle loving from all quarters, especially on the home turf, ruled currently by my mother. She behaves like a wounded lioness instead. She rages on, she despairs, she cares. In that order.

Mothers are most likely human beings. My own demonstrates signs of being made of flesh, blood and feelings. I'll touch forty in a year and this one still chides me, feeds me, overrides me, gets bored of me, shirks me (her perennial responsibility) and often manipulates me. Then she turns around and flings at me a golden web of indescribable love and weaves it tightly all around. From this, there's no escape. For her or me.

Mothers are also dangerous people. Mothers in post-partum depression are known to smother babies. Mothers can take on lovers. Mothers can ambush their blood-sucking dependents by walking off in search of golden horizons. Mothers can be audacious, they can lay claim to their own life. Scorned mothers can be vile and unforgiving.

Mothers have been choking slowly. Five thousand years of our culture has turned them into shrine-worthy goddesses. To be venerated. Prostrated before. All the while, expecting them to radiate gentle goodness in the face of calamities like suffering children, growing dullness in their souls, an acerbic, callous society perennially watching for slip-ups. And after all this, they are cast away in the waters once their season is over.

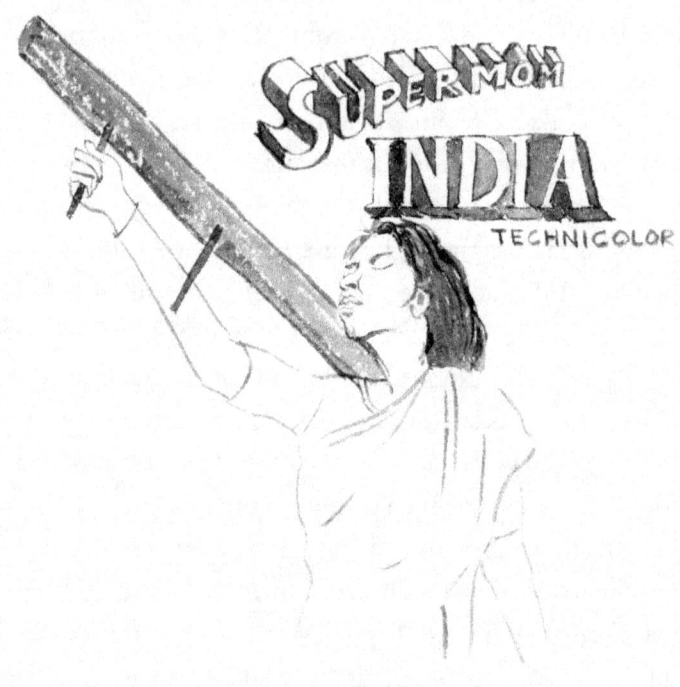

If we must make our mothers into shrine-worthy clay goddesses, let us build them up with a margin of errors. Like a little chink on one shoulder or a minor design flaw; a small structural mistake (like the head slightly out of place); a crack running through the back or some scraping of paint. This will give them breathing space.

Till then, my own will continue to give me heaven and hell for being sickly all my life.

21
The Tall Women

Try as you may, you cannot count my mother and me as tall women. We are decidedly petite though. Midgets, declares the husband.

The tall women in our family are my mother-in-law and sister-in-law. Again, they are not vertically much to write home about, but I mean as people. They have spines of steel, they are unfazed by life's botherances, they retain high spirits and dispense their duties with an infectious smile.

When my mother takes a break from me, she writes out instructions and leaves me in my sister-in-law's care. My brother's wife is about my age but her sense of duty and care is almost motherly. She is also inventive; she stirs up new recipes for my chemo mouth; is fun to hang out with and slips me an occasional drink of chilled beer to pep me up on gloomy evenings.

While in Jaipur, my mother-in-law, teetering with

The Tall Women

arthritis mightily climbs up and down a dozen or more steps to give me hour-long massages. When she extends her magical touch, I am relieved of my debilitating pains. For a while, I can cock a snook at morphine tablets, Fentanyl patches and painkillers.

In my numerous hospital admissions, both have cheerfully stayed the night with me, in not very hospitable conditions. My sister-in-law was even excited that the bunk bed she slept in, next to me, made her feel like we were travelling together in a train. She doesn't know till date that I passed that horrible night with pockets of happiness, thinking of fun train journeys from the past.

Nothing that I know of in the law, binds these two to me. Whoever decided to call them in-laws?

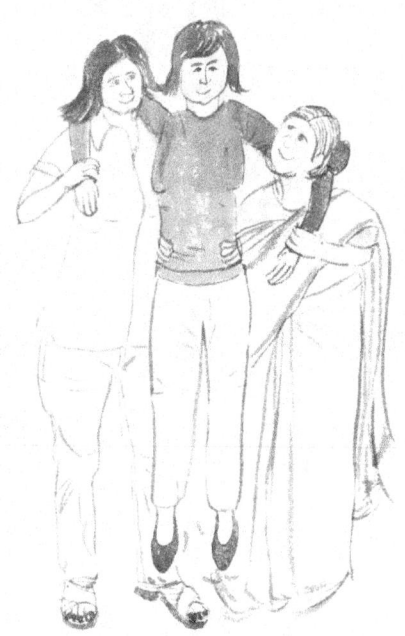

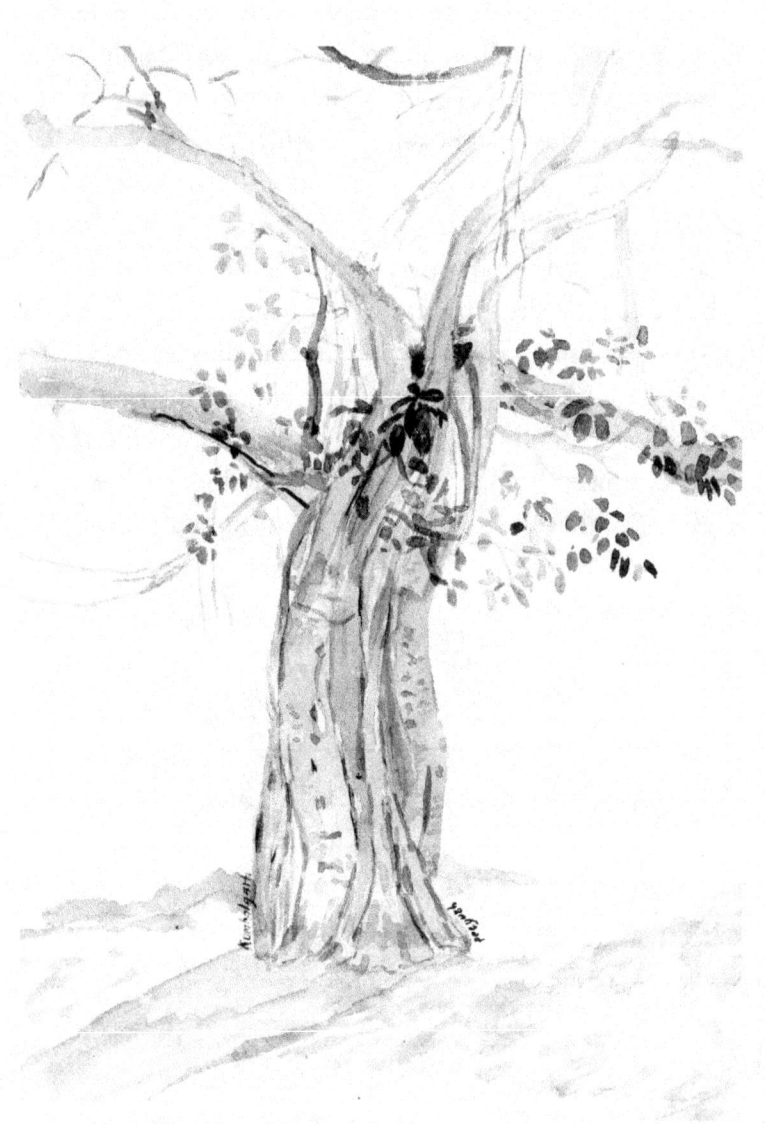

22

Like a Banyan Tree

I have two brothers. One related by birth and the other from another mother. They are like banyan trees. Sturdy, strong with an abundance of compassion for those who seek their shade or want to rest in their branches.

By now, they have been run down by life's many storms. They are not smiling, lush trees anymore. Their trunks look weaker, their branches are bent and leaves brown. Yet I fly to them often, to seek solace from my aches and rest my broken wings a tad.

Rejuvenated, I fly back home again. They don't stop me, they wave me goodbye with their emaciated selves and shower a heap of dry leaves by way of blessings. This happens time and again.

23

Beauty and the Beast

I lived in Delhi for a large part of my life and moved to Jaipur only after acquiring a husband. I couldn't take to the city. To make me like it, the husband tried many tricks, none of which worked. He said one of the city's laurels was topping the Happiness Index among Indian cities, several years in a row. I told him it's happiness seemed to be an outcome of being hemmed in, being constricted.

I told him I don't like the street names—Imli Fatak, Jaleb Chowk, Jhotwara, Jhaalawar, Jhaalana Doongri, Moti Doongri. Awful, they sound. What about Timarpur, Mayapuri, Munirka, Masoodpur, he threw at my face?

I am a fan of the metropolis. I like the pulse of a big city. The glamour, the greed, the opportunity, the violence, the madness and the anarchy. Delhi, Gurgaon, Mumbai, Kolkata have passed my litmus test. (I am suspicious of Bangalore—it is a cross between a cultured *halli* and a drunk, buzzing IT hub.)

Beauty and the Beast

I miss Delhi. Its desi beauty in winters, wrapped in fog. Its burning summers. Falling apart at the seams during the rains. The green of the city's affluent, the brown of the down-to-the-wire, and the yellow haze of everyone else caught in between (like the dull glow of DDA flats in the fading sun). The boorishness of its junta, the discoloured, blank-eyed pigeons on its windowsills. The city's characterless character. Loosely moralled. With no respect for boundaries. Lacking in compunction. Much like myself. Standing tall, stuffed

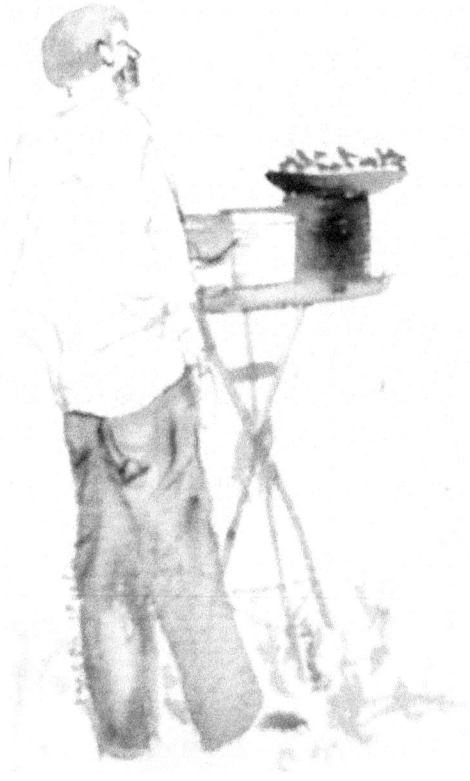

with pride, despite its failings. Yet, grovelling from time to time, to get what it wants. And finally threatening to choke up its very own, in its poison and rancour-filled fumes.

I identify with this beast of a city. In return, the beast loves me back with all it has. With its cosy corners, its secret highs, its superficialities, its fake polish, its seedy underbelly, its wicked smile, its blood, sinew and all.

Jaipur on the other hand, is a beautiful and peaceful city. It seems to have values. Values that are supposed to be good. Family-type values. Extended-family type values. A stable group of friends (who must be family folks too). They keep you grounded (chained, I think). Tethered. Like a farm animal. With a defined grazing radius. Lest you graze too far, run amok, snitch other people's stuff, cause destruction. (In Jaipur, the State Women's Commission is housed along with the Livestock Development Board. Such coincidences are not without reason.)

To me, this city represents a careful confinement. An oppressive pinkness. An unnecessary gaiety of its bazaars. Arches, pillars and havelis stifling you wherever you go. An old-worldliness like a veiled threat: 'Stay old and conventional'. It represents the suffocating safety of long marriages. Elevation to the status of a worthy, virtuous woman if you play by its rules.

In the first few years of my marriage, I spent many days brooding about my detethering. I imagined it would be conscious. Now that it is accidentally

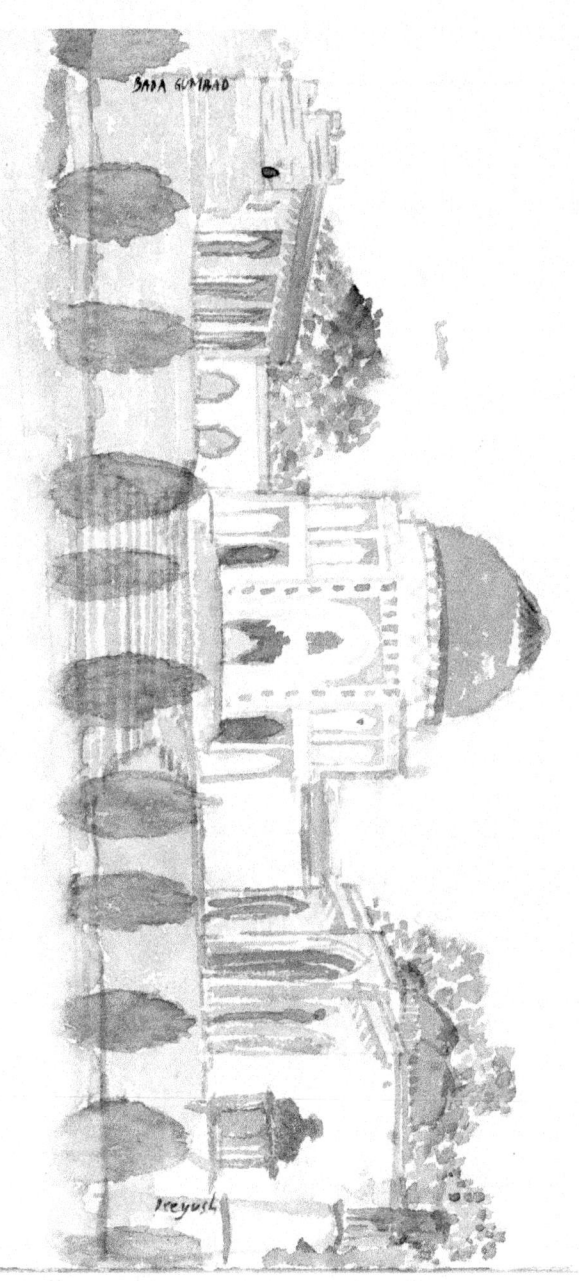

happening, I wonder whose arms I would go to next, given a choice?

A powder blue, dull and safe heaven, that will pat me down to sleep? Or a familiar hell, like an unfaithful, grisly old lover who will keep me awake in a perennial state of brouhaha.

Your guess is as good as mine!

24
Yolo

My friend with the booming voice visits me one early Sunday morning and tells me that the in-thing these days is 'YOLO'. I give her a look of complete incomprehension. She yelps loudly, 'You don't know YOLO?' Drowsy birds enjoying their Sunday morning on my terrace fly away quickly. The dog raises his tail in alarm. And I spill hot tea on my lap. Unfazed, she proceeds to explain, 'YOLO means "You Only Live Once". Hence, you are supposed to live life kingsize, do what makes you happy and have no regrets.'

Impressed with my newfound knowledge, I decide to test the old mate on how clued-in he is, in the same way my friend with the booming voice tested me.

It's a mellow evening, the husband has parked himself on the terrace on a bean bag. He sits dreamily with eyes half-closed, drumming his belly lightly. I yell

YOLO into his ears. He gives me a look of disgust, and drags his seat a few feet away.

Cancer has brought the focus on if I have lived my life well. If have lived my life YOLO. Quite so, I conclude. I have always taken my own decisions, lived life as I pleased, made many mistakes, ill-informed choices and have always been wiser in hindsight. The best part is I have had no one to blame, and faced with the consequences of my actions, I have been quite kind, loving and forgiving towards myself.

The only regret I have is I have been a drifter. Surrounded by well-grounded people who had perfect blueprints for their life ahead, I don't know how I ended up drifting around. People I hung out with had prototypes of dreams. Crafted on butter-paper, rolled up carefully and stored in lockers. A stable life with a decent job and relationship by thirty. Own home at thirty-five. Assorted—children, plants and pets before forty. A trip to Mount Fuji in the August of the year they turn forty-five. A three-tier cake on their tenth anniversary, a photo of which would go on the blue wall behind the TV for everyone to see.

As much as I ached to fit the bill, I realised early on that I was a drifter. Staying put throttled my soul. Tedium made me dull. Drifters can be interesting people, they can take you along floating with them into newer waters. They can be exciting, challenging and fun, and while they threaten occasionally, only rarely do they sink. But they lack one thing. They can't drop anchor. They can't make prototypes on butter-paper and store them for posterity. They lack stillness, they lack the art of accumulation, the art of staying put—strong and rooted, with a bag of compromises and material securities, if you please.

Cancer has healing powers. It seems to have healed the chronic restlessness of my soul. It has taught me to drop anchor. Stay moored. Cling. Grab like a crab.

'It's not cancer. It's age catching up, old girl,' the husband adds by way of extra comments.

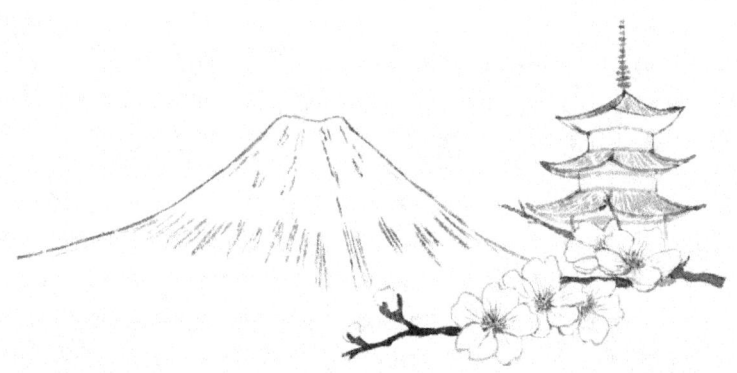

25
Hope As a Strategy

Malcolm Gladwell, the renowned management guru said hope cannot be your strategy. I wonder if it is true.

When I get a chemo break, I return to my in-laws house in Jaipur. I am greeted by a thin green creeper growing forcefully from a crack in the stone wall. I occupy a room on the first floor with a big terrace. My mother-in-law's champa tree stretches its arms up eagerly from the ground floor to touch the terrace. After many an insomniac night spent fighting back pain and other demons, I wake up to see the champa bursting with bright, sweet-smelling flowers, stretching its arms even higher to reach up to me. Its hope is infectious.

Hope out of thin air is magical. It helps forget bitter experiences. On silent nights, it narrates nice new stories where you are the immortal hero, no disease can touch you, success sticks like glue, happiness lasts enough to savour and marriages are more fun than drudgery.

Hope As a Strategy

After a few weeks of relaxing, smelling flowers and checking out the creeper growing merrily out of the stone wall, I head back to Mumbai to resume my treatment.

One day, waiting for a doctor's appointment, I find my father hunched over, comparing my histopathology report with another man, who's showing his wife's. The two semi-bald heads are going over line by line of the reports that are laid out side by side, comparing stages and grades of our respective tumours.

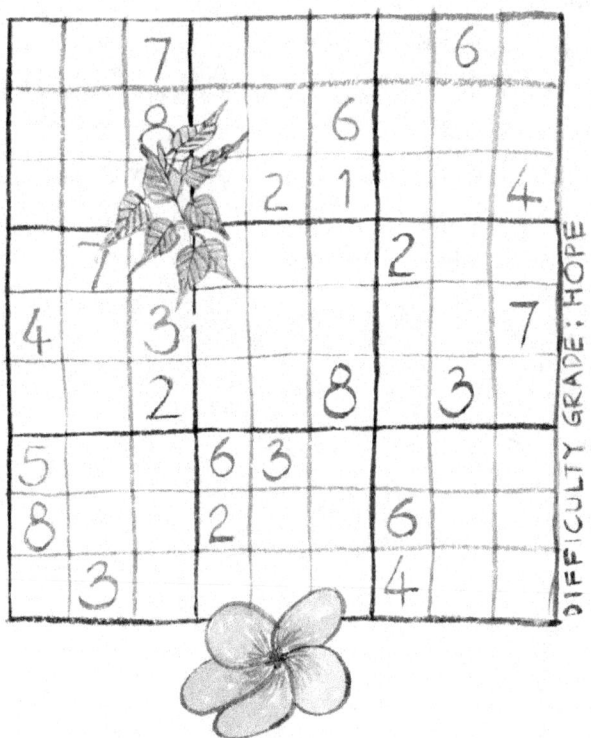

The sight wrings my heart and takes me back to my school days when my dad and other parents used to compare our report cards. The only difference now is he's older, sadder and as a civil engineer hasn't the remotest idea of what he's comparing. But once again, I hope my report card isn't bad enough to embarrass him. Thankfully neither party has any clue of what they're comparing, so there's no verdict of which patient has a better chance of making it through. After a while, they close the files and stare in different directions.

Meanwhile, the days in the metropolis go by. My dad and I wait endlessly at hospitals. Clutching our bagful of medical reports, scans and X-ray films. Doing our sudokus and playing our mobile games. Drinking our coffees silently.

I take after my dad. We are like solid working class people. Heartbreakingly practical and unimaginative. Only this time, hope happens to be our strategy.

26

Fear Is Just a Four-letter Word

I've not known fear. I've never been afraid of pitch dark closing in on me, one-eyed ghosts, shady men, dizzying heights, closed spaces…you name it. The only thing I've been borderline scared of, have been spiders.

Till some time back, my biggest nightmare had been going to empty my bladder, middle of the night, eyes dreamily half-closed, or whistling away, doing my morning job, staring at pictures of pishposh people in *Mumbai Times*, and a vicious, giant tarantula crawls up from its hiding spot under the pot and goes straight for my unsuspecting ass. Needless to say, I'm done for.

Before this fear could come true (thankfully), I landed up in Australia for a year-long project, totally ignorant of the fact that the country boasted of having the most poisonous, most dangerous and largest spiders in the world.

As I struggled to make peace with the red-back

spider, the funnel webs, the trap door ones and the Aussie tarantulas that can eat a bird (my emaciated backside was nothing in comparison, I'd shuddered), one fine day I found a jet black, bushy spider, at least fifteen inches long, sitting still in my bathtub. Okay, I may be exaggerating a little here, but I swear it was no less than five inches across. Spotting it, I promptly let out a shriek, which of course no one heard, banged the bathroom door shut and left for work. In the evening as I opened the door a crack and peeped through, hoping to see the eight-legged black monster enjoying a hot bath, I was surprised that there was no action; the spider lay motionless in the bathtub in the same position as I had left him. This continued for two more days. Bathless for three days and in the grip of a nightmare featuring the damn thing crawling up my bedpost, I peeped morning and evening, only to find the furry intruder waiting for Godot. On Day Four, it struck me that my eight-legged intruder might be dead. Then I thought, what if he was pretending to be dead and the moment I poked him, he would jump at my face and claim his pound of flesh? Crocodiles are known to do this all the time. I reasoned with myself that this was no sly crocodile and in any case, let another couple of days pass before I took action. On the appointed day I put on my favourite music on my iphone on full blast, put my earphones on, shoved the phone in my jersey pocket, took a broom and dust pan and scooped the damn thing on the pan. Just the action of the broom touching the spider made my skin crawl all over. Then I ran outside at full speed with the dust pan, like a crazy woman, and emptied it in the dry grassy patch next door. Easy as that!

My furry Aussie mate had an unprecedented effect on me. From that day on, I started feeling less scared of spiders. I still didn't like them enough to smile at them, look them in the eye or say howdy. But you get the drift.

Presently, that fear has been replaced with another one. In Hinduism, some say that human life is measured in breaths and not years. Each one of us is allotted a certain number of breaths and your end comes when you have exhausted them. Now as I experience shortness of breath or get breathless with just talking fast, this new fear has me in its grip. The fear of my breaths running out. The fear of not being able to breathe. My chest constricts with the thought and I start breathing fast. Then I panic that breathing fast will cut my number of breaths, so I try to breathe slow. My days continue with this tussle.

This morning, sitting on the throne and once again feeding my voyeuristic side with the lives and times of the rich and famous, I see a little spider trying to crawl up a slippery tile in front of me, to reach its web that's hanging just above the tile. Though I am past my arachnophobia, yet I can bet no one would feel scared of this one. It's the Indian variety, scrawny, hungry and in the absence of fur or hair, looks naked and embarrassed of its appearance. As I watch it diligently try to crawl up at least twenty times after slipping down, I'm reminded of the story of King Bruce and the spider that I'd read as a child. The gist of the story was—a defeated King Bruce hides in a cave and is impressed by a spider's relentless efforts to get up and going on a wall. Motivated by the little creature's numerous efforts, King Bruce realizes that giving up is not an option but trying hard is. He goes back to the battlefield and emerges victorious this time.

By the time I remember the full story, my brave little spider has crawled past the tile and is hanging peacefully in its impoverished hammock, sprinkled with dust, enjoying a tiny insect or two.

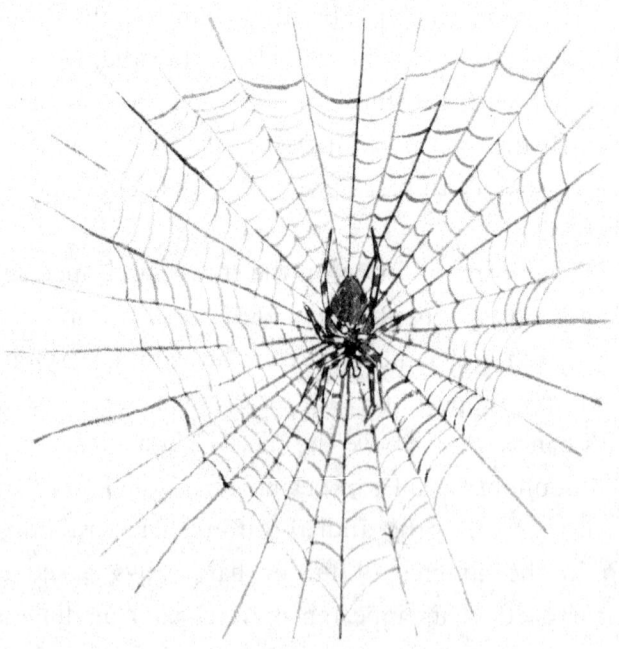

That night as I lie on my bed breathing softly, counting breaths, fighting the fear of my breaths getting reduced, I think of my Aussie demon, the tiny spider in my bathroom and King Bruce's spider in the medieval cave. I need to slay my fears and try one step at a time.

Remember the song from the famous Bollywood flick, *Mr Natwarlal*, where Amitabh Bachhan sings to a group of kids about fighting fear of a tiger in a dense jungle? Because otherwise, *'Ye jeena bhi koi jeena hai, lallu?'*

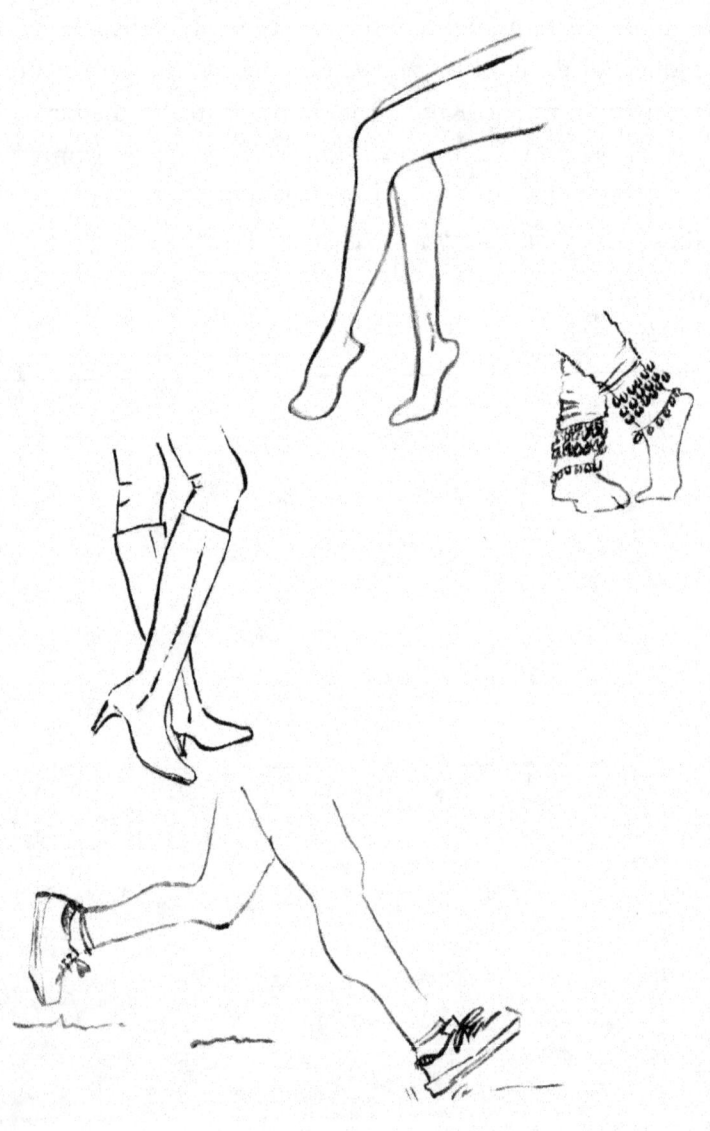

27
These Legs

These legs.
    Give me sleepless nights,
    Ache furiously,
    Scream silently,
    Calm down only after I swallow a handful of pills,
    Sleep fitfully after,
    Sated, in the morning they make me feel beautiful again,
    These treacherous legs.

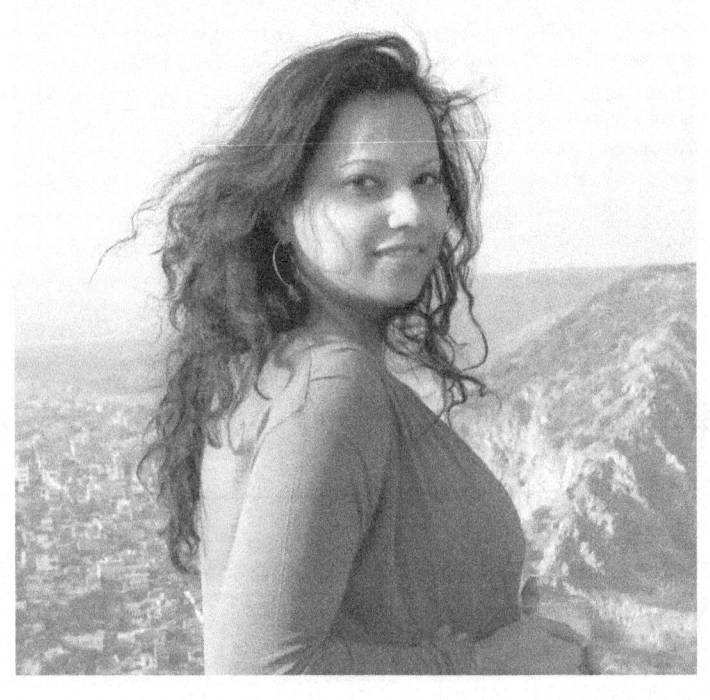

Afterthoughts

'We should get an air cooler instead of this AC. Cooler air is fresh, it's eco-friendly. The air conditioner gives one a sore throat and a headache every morning when one wakes up,' I told Ananya after reading a WhatsApp forward that I had received.

'Sure, and while we are at it, let's dispose of this flat screen TV and get a black and white and also let's get rid of the car and you can buy a Bajaj scooter. Let's live like it's the 1980s. Let's move back a century instead of moving forward,' Ananya retorted.

Sharp wit, quick thinking, lack of pretence and a hyper intelligent mind, that's how I remember Ananya. Of all the faults that she could be accused of, hypocrisy and doublespeak were not on the list. She always walked the talk.

In the year 2000 when we both joined Symbiosis College, Pune, I noticed Ananya almost on the very first day for her humour, gorgeous looks and intelligence. We soon became friends. It was a no-brainer that this girl was way out of my league, so good friendship was the only way forward.

After college, life took us in different directions but we managed to keep in touch through the highs and lows of life. A chance meeting before she was to leave for Australia to pursue higher studies, led to something unforeseen. The articulate, humorous and beautiful girl from Delhi started taking an interest in the smalltown boy from Jaipur. 'If I come back do we have a future?' she asked.

'Sure,' I said without much thought. Who comes back from Australia, I said to myself. But come back she did, in 2010. My Marwari friends have always believed in the adage, 'The wise rush in where fools fear to tread.' This time I acted with haste and wisely, and we got married.

I would like to believe that life was all a bed of roses for her afterwards but the reality is that in one single move, Ananya had said goodbye to her corporate career, six-digit salary, friends, and the life she had built over a decade in Delhi, a city she loved. To her credit she never mentioned this once in our most heated arguments. It was not in her nature to sit and grieve over circumstances. She often said, 'Get up and get to work, Mr Bhasin, that's how you solve problems in life.' Brick by brick, day by day she built everything that she had left behind. A job to keep her busy from nine to six, a small set of friends and a well-furnished home.

The years just flew by and it was time to think

about increasing the size of our family. It was during her medical check up that the doctor noticed a lump in her left breast. She was diagnosed with breast cancer. But there was nothing to worry about, the disease is curable. The support groups, the doctors, the survivors, all said the same thing. We believed that if we followed the doctor's advice, things would be all right. We were all wrong. Ananya breathed her last on 18 November 2018. For perhaps the first time in her life, will did not triumph over circumstances. But as she fought the disease for twenty-two months, she managed to continue her job, including outstation travel, wrote reports for our NGO, Muskaan, devised and managed social media for my business, and wrote a book. She did this while undergoing a major surgery, several intrusive scans, over fifty chemo cycles, sedatives and bearing the excruciating pain. She did what she preached, got up and went to work every day.

A few days before her demise, she mailed a final copy of the manuscript to Ravi Singh at Speaking Tiger. She managed to meet her deadline for this one too.

In the end, what has happened is not what we desired but I do believe that for all the work that she accomplished in a single lifetime, God will relieve her of cycles of reincarnation. I have a basketfull of memories that will sometimes bring tears to my eyes, often make me laugh. Much like this book.

Shantanu Bhasin
Jaipur, June 2019

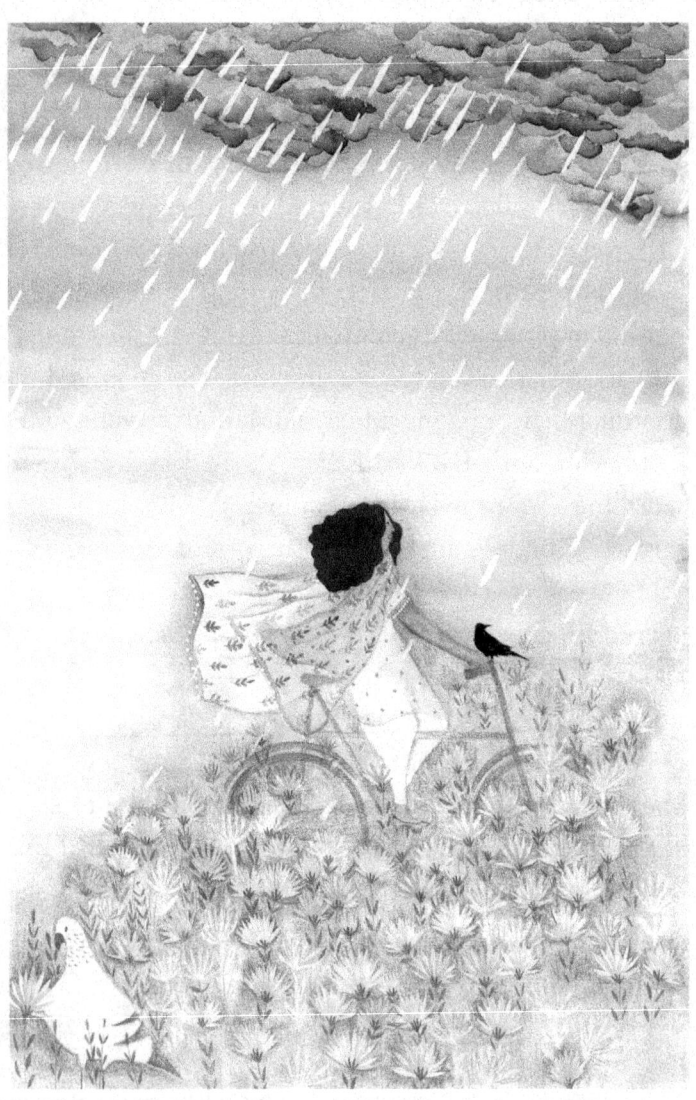